WEIGHT LOSS

THE

JABEZ

WAY

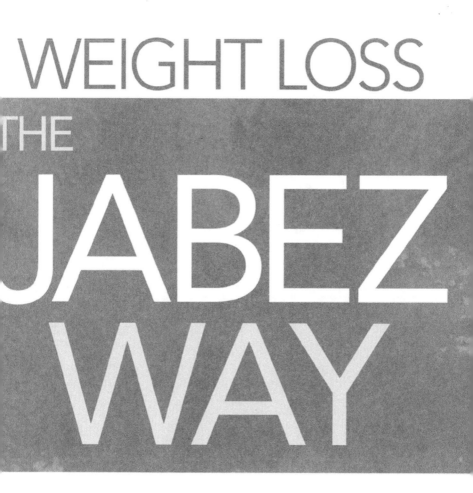

7 Keys to Adding Years to Your Life
& Life to Your Years

SCOTT CONARD, MD

COVER, INTERIOR DESIGN & PRINT PRODUCTION:

Inprov, Ltd.
2150 E. Continental Boulevard
Southlake, TX 76092
www.inprov.biz

EDITORIAL CONSULTANT:
Vincent M. Newfield, New Fields & Company • P.O. Box 622 • Hillsboro, Missouri 63050
www.preparethewaytoday.org

Printed in the United States

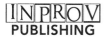

FOREWORD

FOREWORD

BY JAMES ROBISON

There is a growing concern among health experts about the state of our nation when it comes to health and weight issues. Obesity, diabetes and other health-related concerns are on the rise in a nation of fast-food consumers and fast-paced lives which ultimately rob us of one of God's greatest blessings—our health.

While many are constantly on the lookout for the next great diet or exercise plan that promises quick results, my personal physician, Dr. Scott Conard, has provided a common sense solution to weight loss. His approach is an extension of his focus in medicine and with his patients: "I want to help empower you to make good choices about your health."

This is not just another book about dieting, but an approach to healthy living and weight loss, founded on the prayer of Jabez in the Old Testament. *Weight Loss the Jabez Way* allows each reader to think about personal desires and goals and how to incorporate diet, food intake and exercise in the way that is best for them. It is not a "one size fits all" approach to weight loss.

You were uniquely created by God, and as you follow the seven powerful principles based on this powerful prayer, you can develop an effective and personal plan for weight loss and ultimately enjoy a healthier life.

I've known Dr. Conard personally and professionally for many years, and I know firsthand that his passions to help people live longer, live healthy and feel good are at the core of his medical background. I appreciate this medical approach to weight loss coupled with wisdom based on God's Word. This is a very different book on weight loss, because it is designed to direct you and connect you with the Source of all the answers—God. Losing weight, enjoying health and drawing closer to God! Now, that's a plan!

James Robison

President, LIFE Outreach International

TABLE OF CONTENTS

Foreword by James Robison   7

Introduction   15

Chapter 1: Surrender   23

Chapter 2: First Steps   35

Chapter 3: Expanded Horizons   49

Chapter 4: The Seven Healers   61

Chapter 5: Turning Point   75

Chapter 6: Making the Right Choices   91

Chapter 7: A Life of Peace   105

Conclusion   121

INTRODUCTION

INTRODUCTION

Atkins . . . South Beach . . . Weight Watchers . . . Carb Blockers
. . . Jenny Craig . . . The Zone . . . you name the diet, Judy had
tried it. Yet successful, sustained weight loss and improved
health continued to remain just out of her reach. Frustration,
hopelessness, depression and defeat hung over her head like
an ominous black cloud. Our office was her last resort.

"I've tried everything, and nothing works," she said. "My
blood pressure and cholesterol levels are sky high, I have
just been diagnosed with Type 2 Diabetes, my joints are
constantly killing me and I have no energy to do anything.
I don't want to live like this anymore, but I don't know what
to do to change it."

Does this scenario sound familiar? You are not alone. Experts at the Centers for Disease Control and Prevention now estimate that nearly 2/3 of all Americans are considered obese, more than double the amount in 1990. Actually, obesity is such an epidemic that experts are predicting many of the children alive today will have a shorter lifespan than that of their parents.

It may be difficult to admit, but to a great degree, when you stand naked in front of a mirror just before or after your bath, what you see from the *neck down* is a direct reflection of your decisions from the *neck up.* You really can't hate it or love it. It's just like gravity—it is what it is because of what you have chosen to do up to this point in your life. If you keep making the same choices, you are going to keep getting the same results. The question is, what will you choose to do from here on out?

NOW, HERE'S THE GREAT NEWS!

If you are overweight or obese, you don't have to stay that way. You can change! All you need is a willingness to be *open-minded* to the principles presented in this book, not closed-minded because of past experiences. In the world of theater, this is called "a willing suspension of disbelief." In order to successfully move from where you are to where you want to be, you will need to suspend the disbelief or doubts filling your mind, trying to tell you, "You've tried this before, and it doesn't work."

The prayer of Jabez, found in 1 Chronicles 4:10, gives us seven powerful principles to effectively lose weight and live healthy, vibrant lives. Throughout this book, we will examine certain standards and principles of good health proved to be indispensable and true. As we journey, you will be encouraged to apply them to your own life. Your body may or may not respond immediately, and it may not respond exactly the way someone else's does. That's okay.

We could take four people—a post-menopausal woman in her 60s, a mother of four in her mid-30s, a young man with high testosterone levels in his 20s and a man who has little to no testosterone in his 80s—and place them all on the *same diet.* More than likely, we would get four *different* results. The diet may work for one or even two of them, but not all four. And that's okay. The point is, you need to be flexible and try different things until you find the plan that works for *you.*

This book is *not* designed to give you all the answers. It is designed to *direct* you and *connect* you with the Source of all the answers—God. Encouraging you to establish a close, intimate relationship with the Creator of the universe is truly my greatest desire. God has a specific health plan just for you, for *your* age, *your* genetic code, *your* hormone level, *your* metabolic rate, *your* body shape and *your* place in life. Look at what King David says about God:

*(He) satisfies your mouth [your necessity and desire
at your personal age and situation] with good so
that your youth, renewed, is like the eagle's [strong,
overcoming, soaring]!*

—Psalm 103:5 AMP
(Word in parenthesis added for clarity.)

The truth is, *you* don't know what to do to lose weight in a healthy way and keep it off, but God does! The Great Creator of heaven and earth and your own body, knows the way and promises to *instruct you and teach you in **the way** you should go; I will counsel you and watch over you* (Psalm 32:8 NIV).

Are you ready to begin? Are you ready to "suspend your disbelief," putting aside all doubts, fears and preconceived ideas of what has happened before? Are you ready to be open to a whole new way of looking at and living life? Don't let your past predict your future. Be open to the miraculous results you can receive as you entrust yourself to God!

AS YOU BEGIN YOUR JOURNEY OF *WEIGHT LOSS THE JABEZ WAY* . . .

Humble yourself before the Lord and make this your prayer:

*Show me the right path, O LORD;
point out the road for me to follow. Lead me
by your truth and teach me, for you are*

the God who saves me.
*All day long **I put my hope in you.***

—Psalm 25:4-5 NLT

Now *hear* and *hold onto* God's promise to you:

He will teach the ways that are right and best to those who humbly turn to him.

And when we obey him, every path he guides us on is fragrant with his loving-kindness and his truth.

*Where is the man who fears the Lord? God will teach him **how to choose the best.***

—Psalm 25:9-10, 12 TLB

Jabez cried out to the God of Israel, "Oh, that You would bless me and enlarge my territory! Let Your hand be with me, and keep me free from harm so that I will be free from pain." And God granted his request.

—1 Chronicles 4:10 NIV

CHAPTER ONE 1

CHAPTER ONE

SURRENDER

Jabez cried out to the God of Israel . . .

In the brief account of the story of Jabez in the Old Testament, the first and most important thing we see Jabez do is cry out to God for help. Somehow, some way, he came to the place where he realized he needed help beyond human power. Therefore, he turned to one greater than all things, the ultimate source of provision—God.

Similarly, in order to experience real, lasting change in the area of weight loss, you and I have to come to the place where we realize we don't have all the answers. The truth is, if you knew how to lose weight and keep it off, you would have already done it. But you don't have the answers. So you must seek the One who does. God's love for you is immeasurable! He created you and intricately formed you in your mother's womb and knows exactly what you need to do to realize your ideal weight and keep off excess pounds. He will reveal to you the steps you must take, but first you must *surrender* yourself to His care.

> "The greatness of a man's power
> is the measure of his *surrender.*"
>
> —William Booth[1]

NIX BEING A "KNOWER"

Take a pen and a piece of paper, and on the paper, draw a circle large enough to fill the page. Imagine this circle represents all the knowledge there is to know in the entire cosmos—the knowledge that only God, the great Creator, knows. Out of all this knowledge, how much would you say you know? For the sake of this example, let's be generous and say you know 1%. From the center of the circle, draw a very small sliver, or pie piece, representing your 1%. This symbolizes all the data and your opinions about the data that you have accumulated in your life up to this point. Got it? Good.

Of all the remaining knowledge, there are some things that *you know* you *don't know*. You probably don't know Swahili, Chinese or Russian or the names of the children who were born today in the city of St. Louis. But you could go find it out. Yes, it would take time, but you could go online and find the information. My point is, there is another segment of insight that *you know* you *don't know*. For the sake of our example, let's estimate it to be about 4%. With this in mind, carve out a slightly larger sliver of the circle next to your 1%.

So what are you left with? A mammoth amount of information that you *don't know* that *you don't know*—approximately 95%. And within the 95% is the individual, tailor-made plan of action you need to lose your excess weight and keep it off. The question is, how do you access this enormous wedge of wisdom? There is only one way. Just as Jabez came to the end of himself and turned his life over to God, we must do the same. We must surrender our status of being a "knower," thinking we have all the answers, and take the position of a "learner" by leaning on the one who really does know.

> "No soul can be really at rest
> until it has given up all dependence
> on everything else and has been forced
> to *depend on the Lord alone.*
> As long as our expectation

is from other things, nothing but disappointment awaits us."

—Hannah Whitall Smith[2]

BECOME A "LEARNER"

Jesus Christ, the world-renowned Master, Teacher, Prophet and Rabbi who walked the earth over 2,000 years ago, offers you and all mankind a timeless invitation. He says, *Come to me, all you who are weary and burdened, and I will give you rest. Take my yoke upon you and **learn** from me, for I am gentle and humble in heart, and you will find rest for your souls. For my yoke is easy and my burden is light* (Matthew 11:28-30 NIV).

In over twenty-two years of medical practice, I have seen countless people burdened with trying to lose weight. Weary and worn out, they often became trapped in a vicious cycle of losing and gaining. It was only when they truly turned their lives over to the Lord and chose to "learn from Him" that they began to experience life-changing success and find true rest.

What does becoming a "learner" look like? It *starts* with humbly admitting you don't have all the answers and turning your life over to the One who does. It *continues* by developing a new way of thinking—a way of thinking that can best be summed up in the words of King Solomon, one of the wisest men ever to rule:

Trust in the Lord *with all your heart*
and lean not on your own understanding;
In all your ways acknowledge him,
and he will make your paths straight.
Do not be wise in your own eyes;
fear the Lord and shun evil. This will
bring HEALTH TO YOUR BODY
and nourishment to your bones.

—Proverbs 3:5-8 NIV

Without question, this timeless text, which is nearly 3,000 years old, still holds infinite value today. As you live day-by-day, moment-by-moment, trusting in the Lord instead of your own limited knowledge, you have open access to the enormous "99%" wedge of wisdom whenever you need it. Does turning your life over to the Lord mean you will never fall back into old unhealthy habits? No. It just means you have made a solid decision to surrender your life to God and as a part of that decision, you are committed to making choices that lead to losing weight.

If, while you are riding in this new direction, you "fall off your horse," choose to quickly get back up. Don't criticize or condemn yourself or try to place the blame on others. Simply choose to run to God in prayer, just as Jabez did. ASK Him for help; SEEK Him for wisdom in His Word and in prayer and KNOCK on the door of His heart until He answers you. *For everyone who keeps on asking receives; and he who keeps on seeking finds; and to him who keeps on knocking, [the door] will be opened* (Matthew 7:8 AMP).

> surrender—to yield; to give up one's self in the power of another.
>
> —*American Dictionary of the English Language,* Noah Webster 1828

WAVE THE WHITE FLAG

Are you ready to surrender? Are you willing to turn yourself over to the divine designer who has all the answers you need to live a fulfilling, healthy life? He awaits your welcome and wants to help you in every area of your life! Don't be deceived into thinking you can keep doing what you've been doing and get different results. Choose to become a "learner" instead of a "knower."

As you turn your life over to the Lord, turn it over with *expectation*! This is a new day in your life—a day of new beginnings and a whole new way of living. With God directing your path, opportunities abound in every area. *Expect* them. The ancient Hebrew text summarizes this sentiment well:

> ***And therefore the Lord [earnestly]***
> ***waits [expecting, looking, and***
> ***longing] to be gracious to you; and***

*therefore He lifts Himself up, that
He may have mercy on you and show
loving-kindness to you. For the Lord
is a God of justice. Blessed (happy,
fortunate, to be envied) are all those
who [earnestly] wait for Him, who
expect and look and long for Him [for
His victory, His favor, His love, His
peace, His joy, and His matchless,
unbroken companionship]!*

—Isaiah 30:18 AMP

Wave the white flag of surrender. Settle the issue of who is in charge. Then expect, look and long for miraculous things to take place in your life!

"I surrendered unto Him all there was of me; everything! Then for the first time I realized what it meant to have real power."

—Kathryn Kuhlman[3]

PRAYER OF SURRENDER

God, I come to You just as I am. Please forgive me for being proud and thinking I have all the answers to life; I don't. And I don't know what I need to do to lose weight, but thankfully You do. I turn my life completely over to You. I have come to the end of me and the beginning of You. I commit myself into Your care and will do what You tell me to do to lose weight in a healthy way. Teach me how to trust in You, hear Your voice and not lean on my own understanding. You know what's best, and I choose to trust You and be open to what I don't know. In Jesus' name, Amen.

HEART OF THE MATTER:

To find the answers you need and lose the weight you want, turn yourself over to God. Learn to live a life of surrender and expectation as you follow His lead in all you do.

(1) Quotes on Submission and Surrender to God (http://dailychristianquote.com /dcqsubmission2.html, retrieved 8/6/09). (2) Ibid. (3) Ibid.

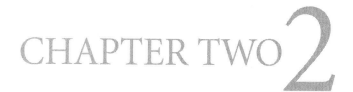

CHAPTER TWO 2

FIRST STEPS

"Oh, that you would bless me indeed . . ."

After Jabez cries out to God for help, he then asks God to bless him indeed. The wonderful thing about losing weight in a healthy, controlled way is that our lives truly are *blessed indeed*! We are not just blessed by a lower number on the scale or our clothes fitting better, but we see our lives made better in every area!

For instance, take "Jay" the truck driver. He came to my office years ago with tears in his eyes, desperately needing to lose weight. His diabetes had escalated out of control, and he could no longer take his medication. If he didn't lose weight, he was going to lose his job and no longer be able to provide for his family. With a stern voice I looked at him and said, "Are you really ready to get serious about this?" He said, "Yes!" So we assessed where he was in his health and established a well-rounded program to help him lose weight in a healthy way.

Amazingly, Jay lost 110 pounds! He went from taking 11 medications a day to taking 2, and that was only the beginning. Not only was he blessed by losing weight and taking less medicine, but his blood pressure went down, his cholesterol level improved and his arthritis got better. Factor in his increased energy, decreased fatigue and all the other benefits, and I think you would agree that God *blessed him indeed*!

As you take your *first steps* to find out where you are, let me encourage you—don't get weighed down by the number on the scale. There are so many wonderful blessings awaiting you, and the greatest blessing of all is the person you will become in the process!

Weight Loss Produces **Blessings** Indeed![1]

- Lower Blood Pressure
- Lower Cholesterol
- Lower Blood Sugar
- Reduced Arthritis Pain
- Reduced or Eliminated Sleep Apnea
- Reduced or Eliminated Heartburn & Asthma
- Reduced the Risk of Cancer, Stroke & Heart Attacks
- Reduced or Eliminated Gout Attacks
- Increased Energy & Mobility
- Decreased Fatigue

"WHERE AM I?"

Just as Jay did, the first thing you must do is find out where you are in your health. Over the years, I have learned that just because a person feels healthy doesn't mean they are healthy. I've seen people come in for what they thought was a simple sinus infection, not even realizing they had sleep apnea, diabetes and heart disease. They were in deep trouble, and all the while they thought everything was "fine."

Situations like these have taught me to dive deeper than the surface symptoms people come in with. If there are any *trouble* spots, we want to find and treat them as early as possible. Using the acronym TROUBLE, my colleagues and

I evaluate specific areas vital to good health. Each of the first six letters corresponds with a *number* related to your current health level. I call them:

THE SIX NUMBERS THAT CAN SAVE YOUR LIFE ™

ONE IS TRAINING.

Training is regular, balanced physical *activity or play*. The number associated with training, a number that can save your life, will vary based upon the level of fitness you are starting from. Counting the number of steps they take each day is a great beginning for those who suffer with significant obesity. On average, people in the United States take about 3,500 steps each day, but for basic health the target is 6,000, about 3 miles for most people. Those really wanting to lose weight should try taking 10,000 steps/day. You can achieve these goals every day by walking, taking the stairs, parking farther away, jogging, doing yard work, playing with the kids, working around the house, dancing and so on.

> HEALTH KEY: Get your *T* in order and be active! Aim for 6,000 – 10,000 steps per day, or if you exercise regularly, get 150 minutes (30 minutes 5 days or 50 minutes 3 days) of activity per week!

TWO IS ROUNDNESS.

Roundness looks at the relation of your Body Mass Index (BMI) to your overall health. If you weigh 200 pounds and are 4'11"as opposed to 6'4", there is a big difference in how you feel and your health. Your BMI evaluates your weight in relation to your height, which you can calculate by dividing your weight by your height (in inches) squared and multiplying that by 703 (go to www.thejabezway.com for a free calculator). Your BMI is the second number that can save your life.

HEALTH KEY: An ideal BMI is 19-25. Determine what BMI is best for you and start aiming toward that goal.

THREE IS OIL.

Oil refers to your *cholesterol levels – LDL, HDL and triglycerides.* While LDL cholesterol and elevated triglycerides can be lethal, HDL cholesterol is actually healthy. An excessive amount of LDL in the blood stream increases the possibility of plaque buildup on the artery walls, and when plaque builds up, arteries become unstable and can break open, leading to a stroke or heart attack.

HEALTH KEY: An ideal LDL is <70; <100 is acceptable. HDL varies by gender—for women >60 is ideal, and >50 is acceptable; for men >50 and >40 are ideal and acceptable. Triglycerides are best kept below 150. To improve these numbers, lower your intake of saturated fats and/or trans fats and replace them with healthy monounsaturated fats (nuts, avocado and olive products).

> "Food is the strongest *drug* you put in your body; exercise is the best *medicine*."
>
> —Dr. Scott Conard

Four is UNACCEPTABLE SUGAR.

Sugar in the form of glucose is one of your body's key fuels (the other key fuel is oil, which we discussed above). The amount of sugar in your body fluctuates naturally within a specific range, according to your food intake, activity and stress level. To keep your sugar level within its normal range, God designed your pancreas to release hormones like insulin into the blood stream. *Unacceptable Sugar* occurs when insulin or glucose levels are either *too high* or *too low* in your bloodstream. These conditions foretell a future of fatigue, diabetes and/or heart disease. So the fourth number that can save your life is your healthy insulin or blood sugar level.

HEALTH KEY: A normal blood sugar level before you eat is between 70 and 100. You can check this in the morning or before you eat. To measure insulin levels, use a test called the c-peptide which has a normal range of 0.5 – 3.2 in most labs, but I believe a level of 1.8 or lower is best.

Five is BLOOD PRESSURE.

Blood Pressure is the force the blood exerts against blood vessel walls. High blood pressure, or hypertension, is a major problem in the U.S., affecting an estimated *one* out of every *four* adults, and is the reason for 10 million office visits a year. It is the forerunner to numerous diseases, including stroke, kidney disease, congestive heart failure and dementia. Although heredity and age, which we can do nothing about, can contribute to high blood pressure, other factors, such as the amount of sodium (table salt) you eat, sleep apnea, exercise and stress levels *can* be adjusted. Your *blood pressure* is the fifth number that can save your life.

HEALTH KEY: Aim for a normal BP reading of less than 120/80 by exercising three to five times a week and adjusting what you eat to foods lower in sodium and higher in potassium.

Six is LOUSY HABITS.

Lousy habits, such as drinking, smoking and taking recreational drugs, kill over 400,000 people a year. Alcohol abuse has been linked to a number of health problems, including heart disease, ulcers and cirrhosis of the liver. Each year in the United States, according to Dr. Stanton Peele, "$10 billion is used to treat people who can't handle their liquor." The cost of drug abuse in America is even higher; researchers estimate it at $67 billion. Amazingly, during the next sixty seconds, *six people* are likely to die from a smoking-related illness.[2] Although the financial cost for these lousy habits is overwhelming, the emotional and social price tags are even greater. The sixth number you need to know is how many cigarettes, pills, alcoholic drinks or hits you are taking daily.

HEALTH KEY: If you're involved in any lousy habits, don't ignore the inevitable consequences that await you. Surrender yourself to God and allow Him and other skilled people help you become blessed indeed.

The last letter in the word TROUBLE is "E" and it stands for *Exploding Plaque* and *Exploding Cells.* While exploding cells are the presence of cancer, exploding plaque is the silent process directly linked to heart attack and stroke. When a catastrophic event of this nature takes place, about half of the victims are completely shocked. Unfortunately, once a person reaches this stage of emergency intervention, treatment options are greatly diminished, which is why it is so important to know the six numbers that can change your life! They will reveal whether or not you're headed for exploding plaque and exploding cells.

HEALTH KEY: Don't wait for your life to explode into an irreversible medical emergency. Take steps now to stay out of *TROUBLE!* Yes, it may take time to get to your goals, but it is worth the effort, *indeed!*

GIVE YOURSELF AS AN OFFERING

So here's what I want you to do, God helping you: Take your everyday, ordinary life—your sleeping, eating, going-to-work, and walking-around life—and place it before God as an offering. Embracing what God does for you is the best thing you can do for him.

—Romans 12:1 The Message

Realize a healthy life will not just happen; it must be created. Are you ready to take your *first steps* and find out where you are in your health? Great! Visit www.thejabezway.com to complete your complimentary TROUBLE report. Remember, being *blessed indeed* goes far beyond seeing a lower number on the scale. Losing weight in a healthy way will affect **every area** of your life. And the greatest blessing of all is the person you will become in the process!

God is so awesome! . . . *by his mighty power at work within us is able to do far more than we would ever dare to ask or even dream of—infinitely beyond our highest prayers, desires, thoughts, or hopes. May he be given glory forever . . . !* (Ephesians 3:20 TLB).

HEART OF THE MATTER: Losing weight in a healthy, controlled way will bless every area of your life indeed! The greatest blessing of all is the person you will become in the process!

Recommended Resources: For a complete discussion of the Six Numbers, to get your TROUBLE report and your free copy of the Dash Diet go to www.thejabezway.com.

(1) Information gathered from: http://weightloss.about.com/library/blhealthbenefits. htm; http://www.webmd.com/diet/tc/obesity-health-benefits-of-weight-loss; http://www.lifeclinic.com/focus/nutrition/losing-weight.asp (retrieved 8-13-09). (2) *Mortality from Smoking in Developed Countries 1950-2000* (published by Britain's Imperial Cancer Research Fund, The World Health Organization, and The American Cancer Society).

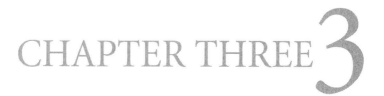

CHAPTER THREE 3

EXPANDED HORIZONS

"And enlarge my territory . . ."

At this point in our journey, we have *surrendered* ourselves to God and are living our daily lives as "learners" instead of "knowers." This position of divine empowerment enables us to stay in our commitment and make choices that lead to healthy weight loss. We have also asked God to *bless us indeed*, which means we are not just focused on seeing a lower number on the scale, but on all the blessings that come from living out our committment to bless and honor the body we have been given, especially the person we become in the process.

Next, like Jabez, we must ask God to *enlarge our territory*. To have our territory *enlarged* means God "increases, expands and broadens" our opportunities on **every** level of life —physically, mentally, emotionally, spiritually, socially, etc. The opposite of *enlarge* is "reduce or decrease," and that is exactly what being overweight does—it decreases our territory, our overall quality of life.

KNOW THE MEANING[1]

Overweight—having a *body mass index* (BMI) between 25.0 and 29.9.

Obese—having a BMI ranging from 30.0 to 39.9.

Morbidly Obese—having a BMI of 40 and above.

Go to www.thejabezway.com to calculate your BMI.
Note: In muscular athletes BMI can overestimate risk.

Body mass index is a value calculated directly from a person's height and weight. To calculate your BMI, divide your weight by your height (in inches) squared and multiply that by 703.

UNDERSTAND THE PROBLEM

Overweight and *obese* are two names for ranges of weight *greater* than what is *generally* considered healthy for a given height. These words also suggest ranges of weight that have been shown to increase the likelihood of certain diseases and other health problems. An adult who has a Body Mass Index (BMI) between 25 and 29.9 is considered *overweight*. One who has a BMI between 30 and 39.9 is considered *obese*.[2] And a person with a BMI of 40 or greater is said to be *morbidly obese*.

Since the mid-seventies, the number of those overweight and obese in the U.S. has increased sharply, both in adults and children. Data from two National Health and Nutrition Examination Surveys (NHANES) show that among adults aged 20–74, the occurrence of obesity increased from **15%** in the 1976–1980 survey to **32.9%** in the 2003–2004 survey.[3] Indeed, obesity has become a major problem in our culture. Sadly, many people don't realize that being overweight not only affects their *quality* of life but also their *quantity* of life, reducing their "territory" of years by as much as decades.

The degree of our obesity is the degree of our DISABILITY; it causes us to "lose or lack ability, immobilize or put out of action." The ultimate disability caused by obesity is permanent: *death*.

Carrying excess weight *shrinks our territory* and disables us from doing many things. It decreases our energy levels, disempowers us mentally and emotionally and diminishes our overall quality of life. For example, a person who is overweight often suffers from joint pain, back pain and muscle aches; they get tired and out of breath quickly, even when doing simple things. Their *territory*, or overall quality of life, is decreased. Can you imagine putting on a 50-pound suit every morning before going to work? How about 100 pounds? How enjoyable would your day be?

This is **not** the way we were meant to live. In John 10:10 Jesus said, *"The thief comes only in order to* steal *and* **kill** *and* **destroy**. *I came that they may have and enjoy life, and have it in* **abundance** *(to the full, till it overflows)"* (AMP). In this case, the thief is excess weight; it steals, kills and destroys our quality of life. But Jesus came to *enlarge our territory*—to give us a full, overflowing and abundant life!

Supermarket Sense

"Spend most of your time shopping the **outside edges** of the grocery store, selecting fresh fruit, vegetables, lean meats, poultry and fish, skim or low-fat dairy products and whole-grain breads. Limit your time in the center of the store; that's where you'll find processed foods that are higher in fat, sugar and salt."

IMPLEMENT THE ANSWER

How is our territory enlarged? God has a part, as do we. We cannot do God's part, and He *will not* do ours. Our part begins by taking the *Six Numbers That Can Save Your Life* and making adjustments in our lifestyles to keep those numbers in healthy ranges. We can make two of the greatest adjustments by *increasing our training* (or play) and *making better food choices* (see Chapter 4).

When we put calories into our mouths, it becomes one of two things: (1) energy or (2) it reappears on our body as fat or lean tissue. The key to success is directing this energy in our body in the right amounts and from the right sources; if we want to get in SHAPE, we need to remember "**S**uccess **H**appens **A**s we **P**rocess **E**nergy."

Processing energy starts with Training, or Play. When our training *increases,* our Roundness, Oil (cholesterol and triglycerides), Unacceptable blood sugar and Blood pressure *decrease.* As you lower these numbers, your body will actually *reverse* the plaque-creating process and begin *absorbing* excess fat out of your blood stream, and lower your risk of Exploding Plague.

Keep in mind that enlarging your territory is not just about losing weight. You could have your leg amputated and quickly lose 25 to 50 pounds or more, but it would not enlarge your territory in a positive way. On the contrary, enlarging your territory is about becoming aware of your body, embracing the Seven Healers™ (Chapter 4) and watching the *Six Numbers That Can Save Your Life* to appreciate your results.

THE "GOSPEL" OF YOUR BODY

You choose what foods you eat; once you swallow the food, you turn it over to the laws God has set up in your body. In this way, studying medicine is studying God's laws after patients have already made bad lifestyle choices and become ill. By getting in touch with the results of your choices processed through God's laws in your body, you can begin turning things over to God a different way and, as a result, experience God's presence in your body and life in a new way. As you walk closer with God, you will make better choices and God will reward you and enlarge your territory. This is how you will truly begin to win the Game of Health.

INVENTORY YOUR TERRITORY

Get quiet before the Lord and ask Him to help you honestly answer these soul-searching questions:

- "What kinds of *foods, activities* and *relationships* **reduce** my territory and *disempower* me from living a quality life?"
- "What kinds of *foods, activities* and *relationships* **enlarge** my territory and *empower* me to live a quality life?"

Pray and ask God for His grace—His supernatural power and ability—to limit or eliminate things that reduce your territory and to *include* and *embrace* things that enlarge it.

MAKE WAY FOR THE MIRACULOUS!

Okay, so what happens when you begin to wake up each morning with more energy? When you no longer fade or fall asleep in the middle of the day? When you can think clearly and your mind is not cloudy or confused? The answer: you are able to do so much more than ever before! Your territory becomes *enlarged,* and you become a new person in every area of your life.

One of the most important areas of our lives God enlarges is in our *thinking.* Proverbs 23:7 declares, "*. . . as he thinks in his heart, so is he*" (AMP). In other words, our thoughts are the building blocks of our actions. As we live in a state of surrender to God, we are no longer confined to our measly 1% thinking; instead, we have access to God's 99% wedge of wisdom. This changes everything—the way we see things, our ability to solve problems and our attitudes toward life in general.

Think about it: when something happens that we never thought possible, we call it a *miracle.* As we stay in our commitment to lose weight in a healthy way, in just a matter of time, miracles begin to take place. Clothes you thought would never fit now fit. Activities you thought you could never do, you can now do. Playing ball with your children, going on a mountain hike with your mate, running a race to benefit cancer patients—all can become a reality. God enlarges **everything** in your life: *"For nothing is impossible with God!"* (Luke 1:37 NIV).

HEART OF THE MATTER: To *enlarge* your territory you must ask God to "increase, expand and broaden" your life in all aspects—physically, mentally, emotionally, spiritually, socially, etc.

Recommended Resources: Go to www.thejabezway.com and watch the video, *Getting in the Game.*

(1) Information gathered from: http://eatingdisorders.about.com/od/glossary/g/overweight.htm (retrieved 8-20-09). (2) Information gathered from: http://www.cdc.gov/obesity/defining.html (retrieved 8-20-09). (3) Information gathered from: http://www.cdc.gov/obesity/data/index.html (retrieved 8-20-09).

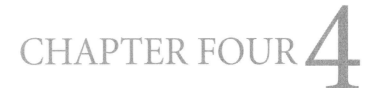

CHAPTER FOUR 4

CHAPTER 4

THE SEVEN HEALERS

"That Your hand would be with me..."

Wow! Things are happening. We are living a *daily* life of surrender to God—we are trusting in Him with all our hearts and not leaning on our own understanding. In all of our ways, including our eating habits, we are beginning to acknowledge Him, and He *is* directing our path. We've also evaluated our TROUBLE spots and begun to make adjustments, especially in the area of *Training. The Six Numbers That Can Save Your Life* are beginning to improve, and slowly but surely we are seeing God enlarge our territory.

As our journey with Jabez continues, we come to the next part of his plea—his heartfelt request for *God's hand to guide him.* What does the hand of God look like? While there is, of course, only one *true* Healer, we can become increasingly aware of His hand in our lives through seven foundational pillars —**the Seven Healers**—*Air, Water, Sleep, Food, Play, Relationships* and *Purpose.* By pulling the Seven Healers into our lives, we experience weight loss and start to enjoy optimum health. Let's take a closer look at each of these incredibly important ingredients.

Simple . . . Yet Profound!

- You can only live about 3 minutes without AIR.
- You can only live 3 to 5 days without WATER.
- You can only live about a week without SLEEP.
- You can only live a month or two without FOOD.
- You will become weak, miserable and sick without PLAY.
- You will feel dead and empty without loving RELATIONSHIPS.
- You will continually fail without discerning your PURPOSE.

THE SEVEN HEALERS

HEALER ONE IS AIR.

Air is oxygen, and every living tissue in your body needs it to live. Did you know that your body removes more waste through breathing than by any other way? If you take shallow rapid breaths, your hands and feet will get cold and you will feel tense and anxious. It takes only 3 minutes of deep breathing to restore a healthy internal balance of air. With 20 minutes of deep breathing, you can significantly alter the stress hormone level of your body and move yourself toward peace and away from stress.

HEALTH KEY: Sit in a comfortable place. Take a deep breath as you say 5, then exhale it to a 5 count as you say "relax" in your mind, repeat this saying 4, relax; 3, relax; 2, relax; and finally 1, relax. Then start at 50. As you breath in say 50, as you breath out say relax; then 49 in, relax out. Continue down to 1. If your mind wanders, no problem, just go back to the last number you remember and pick it up again.

HEALER TWO IS WATER.

Water cleanses and detoxifies your body. Drinking enough every day improves digestion, clarity of thought, mobility, skin health, muscle aches, etc. Are you forgetful or irritable?

Do you have trouble concentrating? These can all be signs of dehydration. To get your body moving in the right direction, drink 8 to 16 ounces of water when you first wake up. When you feel like snacking, try drinking a glass of water instead.

HEALTH KEY: Keep drinking water each day until your urine is clear all the time.

Healer Three IS SLEEP.

During *Sleep,* our bodies and minds rebuild and rejuvenate. Going without it for about a week is a form of torture that leads to temporary insanity. For quality rest, try to go to bed or get up within 15 minutes of the same time each day. Create a relaxing environment in your bedroom: cool, dark and quiet. If you are having problems sleeping, consider removing the television and anything you find that stimulates or produces anxiety. If you choose to drink caffeinated drinks, such as coffee, tea or soda, stop drinking them at least six hours before you go to bed.

HEALTH KEY: Aim for 54 hours of SLEEP each week for optimum health. This is total sleep time —remember that naps count!

Healer Four IS FOOD.

Food is the strongest drug you put into your body. With food that blesses your body, health and wellness ensue. With fatty, sugary and starchy foods, no amount of vitamins, supplements or medication can offset the toxic effects. To prevent cancer, heart attacks and diabetes, eat a wide variety of fresh fruits (2-4 servings/day) and vegetables (5-7 servings/day). Also include whole grain bread and pasta, brown or long grain rice and lean meat. Eat as many veggies as you want, but lean meat should be limited to a serving about the size of the *palm of your hand.* For bread, pasta, potatoes and corn, eat no more than the *height of your fist* and the *width of your fingers* (**with your fingers closed**).

HEALTH KEY: Aim for 50 grams of fiber in your diet each day. Go to www.thejabezway.com and watch the video called "Follow the Food" to become more familiar with this healer.

Power Foods Build Your Immune System and Fight Disease

- Soybeans or Edamame
- Blueberries, Blackberries, Raspberries, Strawberries
- Broccoli, Cauliflower, Asparagus, Cabbage
- Almonds, Walnuts, Macadamia Nuts, Pecans
- Parsley, Tomatoes, Legumes
- Grapefruit, Oranges, Tangerines
- Green Tea

Keep these handy at home and at work. Include them in your snacks. What you buy, you bring home; what you bring home, you eat.

Healer Five IS Play.

Play is Training or exercise that you enjoy! **Exercise is the best medicine for your body**. You were made to move. The less you move, the less you want to move and the less you are able to move. If you were to lie in bed and do nothing, your body would eventually develop fatal blood clots and painful osteoporosis. To keep it going over time find a way to move your body that is fun, enjoyable or rewarding to you. Remember, play doesn't have to be strenuous, all activity counts!

HEALTH KEY: To experience optimum health, PLAY at least 5 days a week for at least 30 minutes. If you are not used to being active, consider getting a pedometer and try to get a minimum of 6,000 steps daily. If possible, make a stretch goal of 10,000 steps for an even greater benefit.

Healer Six IS Relationships.

Relationships are rooted in love, and without love, people die. True friends bring out the best in you (remember, this goes both ways, strive to bring out the best in them). Unhealthy relationships are stressful and actually make you sick. Choose to be in relationships with people who positively support your goals and purposes, and challenge you to grow closer to God and live a healthy life.

HEALTH KEY: Giving and receiving *forgiveness* are the keys to having healthy RELATIONSHIPS. Experience the amazing grace you are given in your relationship with God and express this in your relationships with others (and yourself). Aim to "*. . . always exercise and discipline* [yourself] *. . . to have a clear (unshaken, blameless) conscience, void of offense toward God and toward men*" (Acts 24:16 AMP).

HEALER SEVEN IS PURPOSE.

Discovering your *Purpose* unleashes your motivation for living. It is the "why" behind everything you do, including *why* you get up every day and go to work, *why* you believe what you believe and *why* you want to lose weight and be healthy. Knowing your purpose comes from discerning your gifts and talents and how and where to use them.

HEALTH KEY: Ask yourself this question: "What am I *really* committed to achieving in the next six months to one year?" Write these down on a piece of paper that you keep with you. When you are not sure what to do—take this paper out and ask: "God, what is the best thing for me to do now to achieve this commitment?" Take three deep breaths, calm your mind and see what God sends you as an answer. It could be a thought, a phone call, a person, an email or a knock at the door.

Although *relationships* and *purpose* are listed as the last two healers, they are really the keys to experiencing success in all the others. I have met and worked with people who were "PhDs" in the first five Healers—they understood the importance of Air, Water, Sleep, Food and Play. Yet they weighed over 300 pounds and couldn't lose any weight! Living a life full of supportive relationships and purpose connect and solidify the effectiveness of all Seven Healers.

SEE GOD'S HAND IN IT

The *hand of God guiding you* is seeing your body respond in positive ways to the things it needs most—*the Seven Healers.* As you incorporate these into your life and follow the divine principles of each, you will witness the wonderful effects in your body. Your TROUBLE numbers will decrease, and your "territory" and quality of life, will increase.

If the Seven Healers don't seem to be working, pray and let your body, which is truly the hand of God, guide you in what adjustments you need to make. For instance, instead of being locked into your "1%" and thinking, "It's the Atkins diet that I need," or "I just know the South Beach Diet is the way to go," let your body show you what you need *more* of and what you need *less* of. You have to listen to how your effort with each Healer affects your body and seek to live life from the inside out. No matter how many experts tell you what is right to do by "laying down the law," trust your body, seek the truth and watch Your Numbers—they will direct your energy and help you discover your success.

YOU ARE *FEARFULLY & WONDERFULLY* MADE!

For you created my inmost being;
you knit me together in my mother's
womb. I praise you because I am fearfully
and wonderfully made; your works are
wonderful, I know that full well.

—Psalm 139:13-14 NIV

Fearfully and wonderfully made miracles take place when we embrace the Seven Healers. I have seen many patients experience a dramatic decrease in blood pressure, blood sugar and cholesterol levels. Their bones and muscles grew stronger, sleep apnea disappeared, fatigue faded and energy increased. Fearfully and wonderfully made miracles will take place in you too! Just remember to look for results in the right place—not just on the scale, but in the *Six Numbers That Can Save Your Life.*

HEART OF THE MATTER: The *hand of God guiding you* is seeing your body respond in positive ways to the things it needs most—*Air, Water, Sleep, Food, Play, Relationships* and *Purpose.* As you incorporate these Seven Healers into your life, you will witness the wonderful effects in your body!

Recommended Resources: Visit www.thejabezway.com to access the *Seven Healer Quiz* and see how well you are incorporating each of the Seven Healers.

(1) Jordan S. Rubin, *The Maker's Diet* (Lake Mary FL.: Siloam, 2004, 2005) p. 55.

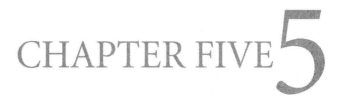

CHAPTER FIVE 5

CHAPTER FIVE

TURNING POINT

"That You would keep me from evil . . ."

Up until now, Jabez's prayer has been focused on God's hand of blessing and guidance. The next request he makes is of a different nature. He asks God to *keep him from evil.* In addition to the spiritual forces of evil we all face at times, *evil* frequently comes to us wrapped in the form of *stress.* In working with patients for over twenty-two years, I have found that the effects of stress depend more on a person's response to the stress than on the stressful circumstance itself. Suppose two people have been diagnosed with diabetes. One will use this as the motivation to re-invent his life, while the other will give up and resign himself to further weight gain, higher sugars and significant complications. They are both facing the same circumstance, but with different *perspectives* that will affect the rest of their lives.

The same principle applies to people's response to the stress they experience as they work to lose weight. When it comes to losing weight, stress can take on many forms, but all of them have one objective—to get you out of your commitment and back on the path of unhealthy living. Your choice, both in those moments of overwhelming stress and throughout your continued journey to health, is whether to overcome the attacks or to succumb to them.

> stress—pressure, strain; a force that tends to distort a body; a factor that induces bodily or mental tension.[1]

Take "Lorraine" for example. She has turned herself over to God and is working to improve her TROUBLE numbers by incorporating the Seven Healers into her life. But after four or five weeks of sticking to her commitment, she still doesn't see the kind of results she wants when she steps on the scale. A few of her friends at work see her disappointment and begin making comments like, "Do you really think it's working? Why don't you go back to the diet you did the last time you lost weight?" Three days later, another friend says, "I think what you're trying to do is great, but don't be such a fanatic about it. Come on; let me treat you to lunch at the Boardwalk Buffet. You need a break!"

A whirlwind of emotions begin to swirl in Lorraine's soul, filling her head and heart with doubt, fear, anger, frustration, criticism and condemnation. In this moment, *evil* is coming against her, and she has reached a *crisis point.* How she responds will determine whether she moves toward or away from success in healthy weight loss.

ADDRESSING A CRISIS POINT

Throughout our lives, we all experience a number of *crisis points*—stressful situations like Lorraine's—when we make choices that become a *pattern* of response for future stressful situations. Some crisis points are more critical than others, but inevitably they have the possibility of pulling us back into learned habits of behavior that will result in another cycle of failure. One of our biggest crisis points takes place during childhood and is directly linked to our relationship with our parents. As we grow, our parents correct us again and again, telling us "No, don't do that. Stop that." Usually before age 4 or 5, we receive their correction at face value and do our best to obey our parents' correction. Then, at some point in our unfolding development, the "No" we heard countless times before has a more profound effect on us. Instead of just receiving their words as correction, we receive them as a *rejection.*

In that moment, an internal panic wells up. Unconsciously, we begin to think things like, *What if Mommy doesn't love me? If I'm not careful, she might send me away.* Or, *Daddy is mad at me. He might leave because of me. What can I do to make him happy?* We do things in an effort to restore peace or regain acceptance. Let's say we clean our room. An hour or two goes by, and we go to them and say, "Daddy, Mommy, look what I did!" They see it and respond, "Oh, baby, that's beautiful. We're so proud of you!" In that moment, peace and acceptance are restored. Now when we feel our parents' disapproval, our "will" (pattern of behavior to experience success) sets in and we do the same things that got us positive results before. In effect, we are setting up a "winning habit," or way of dealing with stress, which we will resort to again and again in our lives in an attempt to overcome our challenges.

One of my colleagues experienced this very thing in her life. When her parents had a second child she was 3 years old. Suddenly she went from being the center of attention to feeling almost forgotten. One morning she, her brother and her mother were at the breakfast table eating their food. Her brother was a finicky eater, and in an attempt to get him to eat, her mom said, "Look at how well your sister eats her food: we never have to make her eat. This makes Mommy and Daddy *so very* happy." In that moment she figured it out. She would eat and please her parents. She did, again and again. In fact, whenever she felt anxious or forgotten, she would soothe her hurt feelings with food.

Forty years later, at over 240 pounds, she attended a training and development course* and discovered this deep-seated pattern of coping. In that moment, she was able let go of food as a way of overcoming her stress and anxiety. As a child, she had made eating a core winning formula for overcoming stress and loneliness. When she let this go and embraced other, more direct and effective ways of addressing her stress, she quickly lost weight. In just over six months, she dropped over 60 pounds, took up dancing and began dating for the first time in a long time.

In our teenage years, a different crisis point takes place, this time, directly linked to our desire to fit in with our friends and peers. This is followed years later by yet another major crisis point, linked to our ability to successfully make it on our own—independent in the world. In these periods of our lives, as we face very stressful situations, we search for winning formulas or strategies to answer core questions like: *What can I do to be accepted? How can I survive in the world on my own?* The actions we take to gain acceptance and cope in the world become unconscious patterns of behavior, locked in as our response when we face additional stressful situations. Literally, in the moment of a crisis, *our will* kicks in and we repeat our past patterns of dealing with stress. Not surprisingly, we set ourselves up to get exactly what we have gotten before when, confronted by stress, we turn to the same tools of survival.

What do these patterns of behavior look like in your life? The answer is literally right in front of you. What do you do when you experience a crisis of stress? If you are overweight, most likely you eat, not because you are hungry, but because this is part of your winning formula. Some of us revert to humor to lighten the stress; others withdraw into books, computers, the TV or other sedentary behaviors. Over time, this withdrawal can turn to alcohol, drugs or obsessive behavior. One thing is clear: what we usually *don't* do is stop and choose a different path in our lives. We turn to *our will* and hope for a different outcome—not a formula usually destined for success.

OVERCOMING A CRISIS: DEFEATING PERCEIVED FAILURE & CONDEMNATION

Going back to our story about Lorraine, let's say she responds to her crisis by accepting the invitation and going to the all-you-can-eat Boardwalk Buffet. As you might expect, when she comes home that evening, she is full of condemnation and self-criticism for what she did. All kinds of negative thoughts are flying through her head: *I'm such a fool. How could I have done that? I'll never succeed. I'll never be able to lose this weight. Every time I start to get a little bit ahead, I do stupid stuff like this.* Lorraine is now dealing with one of the biggest evils imaginable—her internal voice of condemnation and criticism.

This is not the first time this has happened. In fact, as you can imagine, this is what usually happens when she goes on a diet. The more upset she gets, the more stress builds up and the more she turns to her winning formulas for success. Soon she finds herself right back where she began.

It is time for a new way, time to say, "Not my will be done, but *thy* will be done." Silence every condemning voice through *prayer*. Turn to God and repeat to Him in your own words, "Oh, that You would bless me *indeed* and enlarge my territory, that Your hand would be with me and that You would *keep me from evil*. Lord, what I did took me a different way. I am back in on my commitment to you; I want to find the truth, light and way you desire for me. Apart from You I can do nothing, but through You I can do all things" (see John 15:5 and Philippians 4:13). This redirects you back to a humble position of surrendering your will, and in this position you are "in Christ," under His protection, surrendered to His will, free from the cycles of failure you have put yourself through so many times and ready for a new way of living, discovering your true destiny. *There is therefore now no condemnation to those who are in Christ Jesus, who do not walk according to the flesh, but according to the Spirit* (Romans 8:1 NKJV).

Like Lorraine, you are going to go through times on your journey when you fail; you're going to revert to your old habits and overeat, eat the wrong things, stop exercising, lose yourself in your computer, book or favorite TV show, hang out with the wrong crowd, you name it. But just because you fail doesn't mean you are a failure. Think about it: We would say that a *perfect* hitter in baseball is "batting a thousand," but perfect hitters don't really exist. The greatest batters of all time usually have a batting average of around 300. This means that 70% of the time, "the best of the best" fail to reach base. You could say they are "failing" at the plate. Yet in succeeding 30% of the time, they achieve their goal. Remember, you are fearfully and wonderfully made. You don't have to bat 1,000 or even 300 to win with your weight. In fact, it doesn't matter how often or in what way you fail, it matters what you do *when* you are tempted and/or fail. Will you turn to your own will, your own ways, the "winning habits" that got you where you are today? Or will you try a new, different way? King Solomon, one of the wisest men to ever live, said:

. . . for though a righteous man falls seven times,
he rises again, but the wicked are brought down by calamity.

—Proverbs 24:16 NIV

Like a child who is learning to walk, you are learning to walk toward optimal health, and during times of learning, you are going to fall. Just as a child discovers how to balance and successfully move on two feet, you too will discover balance as you stumble toward a healthy life, as you embrace the Seven Healers and as you begin to walk a new way. Don't focus on the fact that you have fallen; focus on how quickly you can get up and get back into your commitment.

KEEPING US FROM EVIL

What is the proper way to respond when we are challenged with stressful situations? How can we overcome our natural inclination to reach into the 1% we "know" to do and do what we've done so many times before? The answer: turn to God in prayer. In that stressful moment when doubt, fear, anger, frustration, condemnation and rationalization all come against you, directing you back into your old way of doing things, turn and run to God instead! In turning to prayer and to His will, you will begin to forgive yourself (and others) quickly and turn back to your commitments. The muscle to make this shift will soon become strong and you will experience yourself through Christ, as the glorious creation you are. This is Him standing with us, allowing Him to provide the strength in our moments of greatest need to take us into the 99% He knows and we don't, and to *keep us from evil!*

In an odd way, the times of greatest stress are our greatest opportunities to grow closer to God. Instead of running *from* stress or suffering through another round of our "winning" habits, we can learn to stop avoiding and running from them. We can "pull stressful situations to us" and have them work to our advantage. Give God a chance to show us a different way, one that will give us freedom and spontaneity in our lives. As we work to strengthen our new muscle, we will begin to avoid old habits altogether. Eating a Big Mac at McDonalds, buying the supersized bag of M&Ms, sitting in front of the TV and snacking instead of going for a walk and exercising—they no longer have power over us. Through Him, we no longer wrestle with the temptations of the evil seeking to defeat us. In our new-found wisdom we win; we just don't go there.

In the book of James, God makes two powerful promises to help us when we turn to Him. He vows to give us *wisdom* on what to do and the *power* of His Spirit to do it!

> *If you want to know what God wants you
> to do, ask him, and he will gladly tell you,
> for he is always ready to give a bountiful
> supply of wisdom to all who ask him; he
> will not resent it.*

> **—James 1:5 TLB**

> *But He gives us more and more grace
> (power of the Holy Spirit, to meet this
> evil tendency and all others fully). That
> is why He says, God sets Himself against
> the proud and haughty, but gives grace
> [continually] to the lowly (those who are
> humble enough to receive it).*

> **—James 4:6 AMP**

As we humble ourselves and turn to God for help and strength instead of arrogantly leaning on our own will and understanding, He will give us the help and strength we need. When we reach a crisis point like Lorraine did, we can turn to God and pray, "Lord, show me what to do. I am overwhelmed, and I feel like throwing in the towel. I don't want to exercise. I just want to eat whatever I want. But in my heart, I know that's not the answer. Please give me grace to overcome the *evil* tendency to go back to my old patterns of behavior. Help me stay in my commitment to lose weight the healthy way. I know You are producing "fearfully and wonderfully made" miracles in my body and in my life. In Jesus' name, Amen!"

HEART OF THE MATTER: *Keeping yourself from evil* is turning to God in prayer the moment you come to a crisis point. When the stress of any situation begins to overwhelm you and you feel yourself going back to your old ways, stop, take a deep breath, pull out your goal list (see Chapter 4) and pray. Then ask God for wisdom as you seek to honor your commitment. You will feel your body calming and your mind refocusing.

Recommended Resources: To learn more about the course referred to in this chapter,* go to www.landmarkeducation.org. The Curriculum for Better Living is a highly-recommended three-course training and development program that begins with the Landmark Forum.

(1) *Merriam Webster's Desk Dictionary* (Springfield, MA: Merriam-Webster, Incorporated 1995).

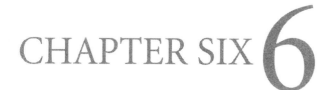

CHAPTER SIX 6

CHAPTER SIX

MAKING THE RIGHT CHOICES

"That I may not cause pain!"

The last request Jabez makes is that he *may not cause pain.*
The truth is, if we are overweight or obese, we are causing
ourselves *and* others a certain amount of pain through
the lifestyle we are living. There are so many ways we can
cause pain, but one of the greatest is missing out on being
a meaningful part of other people's lives. As a result of
unhealthy living, disease can *disable us,* or worse, cause us
to die prematurely. In either case, we are going to cause our
spouse, children and family a lot of pain. This is the pain we

want to be free from, and it really all comes down to making choices that have the Seven Healers active in our lives.

THE *CHOICE* THAT STARTED IT ALL

Without question, the *choices* we make don't just affect us—they affect everyone connected to us. Think back to the beginning of time and the biblical account of the first man and woman, Adam and Eve. God created an awesome world of wonder for people, the crown of His creation, to enjoy. Everything was perfect, from the air they breathed to the food they ate. He gave them full reign and rule over everything. There was only one thing they were not to do: *eat* the fruit from the Tree of the Knowledge of Good and Evil.

You know what happened. They made the *wrong choice* to disobey God and eat the forbidden fruit. The consequences of their choice were devastating, and they aren't the only ones who had to suffer for it. Their choice affected all mankind throughout all generations, including yours and mine. Through their choice, sin and death entered the world,[1] not only affecting humans, but animals, the atmosphere, vegetation and the earth itself.[2] Indeed, this is probably the most powerful example of how our choices can cause pain. And just think . . . all the messy side effects of sin are consequences of a choice connected to *food*.

> "In every decision before us, there is a wise way to go and a foolish way to go—a choice that leads to life and a choice that leads to death. . . . As we spend time in God's presence, feed on His Word, and obey His commands, our lives will be blessed."
>
> —Joyce Meyer[3]

UNHEALTHY CHOICES LEAD TO *DEATH*

Just as there are fruits of *life*—peace, joy, contentment, love, unity, health, etc.—there are also fruits of *death*—strife, bitterness, discontentment, violence, sickness, disease and so forth. I think we would all agree the fruits of death cause great pain. When we consistently make unhealthy choices, we actively plant seeds for the fruits of death, causing a varying degree of harm and pain in our lives and others.

For instance, what happens when "Susan's" choice to smoke results in lung cancer that takes her life in her mid-fifties? How will her destructive behavior pattern affect her two sons, or even the grandchildren born after her death? How about "Roy" whose obesity, resulting from poor food choices and no exercise, leads to heart disease that takes his life in his early sixties. How much pain do you think his widow and three children are dealing with? Or what about "Rachel," a single mother of two whose unhealthy eating, drinking and life of isolation lead to diabetes, high blood pressure and severe depression. Do you think her choices have caused pain to her parents and children?

Unfortunately, the list of stories like these is endless. Undoubtedly, you know a few. The people impacted most by the choices we make are those closest to us, especially our family members. How many times have you been in a restaurant and seen overweight parents sitting with overweight children? As the old saying goes, "The fruit doesn't fall far from the tree." In most cases, kids instinctively pick up the habits of their parents—whether good or bad. Proverbs 10:17 clearly confirms this principle:

> *He who heeds instruction and correction is*
> *[not only himself] in the way of life [but also]*
> ***is a way of life*** *for others. And he who neglects*
> *or refuses reproof [not only himself] goes*
> *astray [but also] causes to err and **is a path***
> ***toward ruin*** *for others* (AMP).

Wow! What eye-opening words of wisdom. If we neglect or reject instruction, in this case regarding healthy living, our lives become *a path toward ruin for others*. However, if we heed instruction and put it into practice, we become *a pathway of life*. As an overweight person, you have an amazing opportunity to bless your spouse, your children, your friends and your community by surrendering yourself to God and wholeheartedly putting these health principles into practice. When you lean on the Lord and receive His grace to live a healthy life, you will teach volumes to others without saying a word!

HEALTHY CHOICES PRODUCE *LIFE*

Just as unhealthy choices produce death in our lives and the lives of others, healthy choices produce life. For me, the greatest example of this is my grandfather. He was a Methodist missionary to India for thirty years and spent his life eating whole grains, fresh vegetables and lean meats, and hiking in the Himalayan Mountains. Because of the healthy lifestyle choices he consistently made, his "territory" was enlarged, God's hand was with him, he was kept from evil and he caused very little pain to others. His life was *blessed indeed*, and I had the joy of living with him all the way into his 96th year!

What would life have been like had he chosen the path that so many people choose today? More than likely, his vitality would have deteriorated in his fifties or sixties, disabilities would have set in during his early seventies and the flame of his life would have been extinguished by his eighties. This would have robbed me of so much quality time with him. I would have barely known him, which would have hurt me greatly, as well as many others. How painful it is for so many who are confined to their couches or can only sit on their front porch, remembering the things they *used to do* with family and friends.

Thankfully, for my grandfather, quite the opposite took place. In my formative years, my grandfather was there with me, active and alert. He challenged and encouraged me to explore the world and embrace other cultures and views, looking for God's guidance in all things. Following the healthy lifestyle principles we have been talking about, my grandfather changed my life. The lessons he taught me through his example frame the person I am today.

"This day I call heaven and earth as witnesses against you that I have set before you life and death, blessings and curses. Now choose life, so that you and your children may live! Choose to love the Lord your God and to obey him and to cling to him, for he is your life and the length of your days. . . ."

—Deuteronomy 30:19-20
[Verse 19 taken from NIV; verse 20 from TLB.]

IT'S ALL ABOUT RELATIONSHIPS

The greatest pain we can cause someone or experience ourselves is within relationships. It is also the place where we can experience the greatest pleasure. Through the loving support of our family and friends, we can learn to make choices that lead to life instead of pain. As Proverbs 11:14 proclaims, *Where no guidance is, the people fall, but in the multitude of counselors there is safety* (AMP).

Let's say you have a really good friend who is trying to lose weight and stay committed to a lifestyle of healthy choices. Sooner or later, they will encounter a very stressful situation —a crisis point that threatens to push them out of their commitment. How would you feel if, in their hour of greatest need, they chose *not* to come to you for help and encouragement? What if they *did* come to you?

The truth is, if someone considered you their good friend and they chose *not* to come to you when they needed help, it could make you feel painfully inadequate. But if they *did* come to you when they were in trouble, it would be a blessing, giving you a sense of value. Now, switch places—put yourself in the place of the person in crisis. Do you confide in others when you're stressed and feel like abandoning your commitment? Or do you choose to suck it up and handle it on your own?

God has designed us to *need each other.* Our family and friends are there to bring out the best in us, and we are meant to bring out the best in them. Sharing our struggles with each other is actually part of the healing process; it's a major key to releasing God's dynamic power.

*Confess to one another therefore your faults
(your slips, your false steps, your offenses,
your sins) and pray [also] for one another,
that you may be* **healed and restored** *[to a
spiritual tone of mind and heart]. The earnest
(heartfelt, continued) prayer of a righteous
man makes tremendous power available
[dynamic in its working].*

—James 5:16 AMP

Confessing our faults and slips is a humbling thing, but the humble are the ones who get God's help, not the proud (see James 4:6; 1 Peter 5:5). When we make the choice to be transparent and share our situation with a trusted friend, we empower them and bring them *pleasure* instead of pain and we get healed in the process!

"I used to do a considerable amount of counseling, and if there's one thing I learned from those interactions, it's that our relationships very often define who we are and what we can become."

—John C. Maxwell[4]

THE CHOICE IS YOURS

Remember, wisdom is choosing to do today what you are going to be happy with later on. The way to bring the least amount of pain to yourself and others is to live a life of surrender to God and obediently follow His leading in everything you do. Are you going to make the right choice every time? No. But if you are living a life of surrender and staying in your commitment, even your failures can become powerful teaching tools for your children and those around you!

HEART OF THE MATTER: Being overweight or obese causes pain to us and others, primarily because it keeps us from being able to participate in their lives in a meaningful way. In order to *not cause pain*, first receive God's grace, then be willing to support others and receive their support in return to consistently make *right choices.*

(1) Check out Romans 5:12-19 and 1 Corinthians 15:21-22. (2) Check out Romans 8:19-22. (3) "Making Right Choices," Joyce Meyer, *Enjoying Everyday Life* magazine, October 2004 (Joyce Meyer Ministries, Inc., Fenton, MO) p. 16. (4) "Relational Refueling," Dr. John C. Maxwell, *Enjoying Everyday Life* magazine, June 2005 (Joyce Meyer Ministries, Inc., Fenton, MO) p. 19.

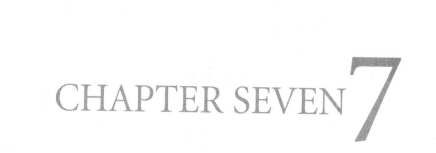

CHAPTER SEVEN 7

CHAPTER SEVEN

A LIFE OF PEACE

"God granted him what he requested."

The final portion of Scripture concerning Jabez's prayer is the acknowledgement that *God granted him what he requested.* Now stop and think about that for a moment. We are living surrendered to God by embracing the Seven Healers and making right choices that keep us in our commitment to lose weight in a healthy way. What would life be like to have God grant us our request? I believe one of the greatest confirmations is experiencing *a life of peace.*

LEARN TO "BE" INSTEAD OF "DO"

A life marked by peace is one that is focused on *being* instead of *doing*. Most people believe that they must first DO something in order to HAVE something; then they can BE what they want to be. As a result, they live their lives constantly rummaging through the "1%" of what they know and trying to figure everything out. I can tell you from firsthand experience that this is *not* a peaceful life.

A life of peace is gained and maintained through a life of surrender. As we turn ourselves over to God, our lives become focused on BEING in Him. We abandon *our* agendas and *our* plans and accept His. To BE in Him is to stand in our commitment; we are not leaning on our own understanding or trying to force things to happen in a certain way or at a certain time. As a result, we gain access to the "99%" wealth of wisdom that only God knows, opening doors of new opportunities, new relationships and new possibilities we never would have experienced if we were relying just on the "1%" of what we know.

As we learned earlier, *prayer* is the key to helping us stay in our commitment. As we dwell in this humble position of surrender, God will show us what to DO. When we find ourselves in a situation where we don't know what to do, we need to stop and cry out to Him for direction, and as we wait upon Him, He will answer. Isaiah 30:21 says, *And your ears will*

*hear a word behind you, saying, **this is the way;** walk in it . . .*
(AMP). Even if it seems like there is absolutely no way out, if
we wait upon the Lord and don't turn back to our *old way* of
thinking, He will make a *new way!*

> *Do not [earnestly] remember the former*
> *things; neither consider the things of old.*
> *Behold, I am doing a new thing! Now it*
> *springs forth; do you not perceive and know*
> *it and will you not give heed to it? I will*
> *even **make a way** in the wilderness*
> *and rivers in the desert.*

—Isaiah 43:18, 19 AMP

As a believer, this is what it means to be "led by the Spirit"
of God. When we are led by Him, we know what to do and
miracles begin to occur in our lives and the lives of others.
Things that we never thought or dreamed were possible
become possible when the hand of God is upon us.

> Consciousness—awareness;
> the quality or state of being aware especially
> of something within oneself.[1]

BE CONSCIOUS OF GOD'S SPIRIT

When we live a life of peace, we discover what it feels like to live free from *self*-consciousness. To be self-conscious is to constantly be *aware of* and *focused on* "self"—what *we* want, what *we* think and how *we* feel. This includes being conscious of our body, focusing on all the physical stimuli we are seeing, hearing, smelling, touching and tasting. Likewise, it also includes being conscious of our soul, focusing on the voice(s) in our head constantly trying to analyze and figure out what we *should* and *could* do or say in the situations we find ourselves in.

Interestingly, the Bible defines this *self*-focused consciousness as the *mind of the flesh*. Romans 8:5 paints a very sobering picture of the mind of the flesh, and it isn't a pretty one:

> *Now the mind of the flesh [which is sense and*
> *reason without the Holy Spirit] is death . . .*
> *But the mind of the [Holy] Spirit is life and*
> *[**soul**] **peace** [both now and forever].*

—Romans 8:6 AMP

So if we are conscious of self, our lives will experience the fruits of death. On the other hand, when we choose to focus on the "still small voice" of God's Spirit living in our spirit, we will experience the fruits of life and peace. Oh, our five senses and our soul are still eager and willing to chime in and tell us what we "woulda, coulda and shoulda" done, but we learn to choose to be conscious of the voice of the Spirit *first* and then receive the other input we need.

For example, you are probably sitting in a chair right now, your body leaning against the chair and your feet touching the floor. Your senses are still sending signals of what is going on; however, you are not consciously aware of it—you have chosen not to focus on it and instead focus on the message God is communicating to you through this book. As you learn to choose to focus on the voice of God's Spirit first, you will experience a life of peace.

> "Self-consciousness is the first thing that will upset completeness of the life in God, and self-consciousness continually produces wrestling . . . It is never God's will that we should be anything less than absolutely complete in Him. Anything that disturbs rest in Him must be cured at once, and it is not cured by being ignored, but by coming to Jesus Christ. If we come to Him and ask Him to produce Christ-consciousness, He will always do it until we learn to abide in Him."
>
> —Oswald Chambers[2]

UNDERSTAND THE VOICE OF YOUR CONSCIENCE

Okay, so how does all this apply to our everyday lives? I think we can best answer this question by performing a hypothetical experiment. Let's pretend "Mary" is on her way to work and stops in at Starbucks to get something to eat and drink. As she walks in the door, we have a special device that enables us to hear the voice of her conscience, detecting all the internal dialogue she is hearing within her. What do you think we might hear?

Scenario 1: "Monkey Mind"

If Mary is focused on the *voice of her soul*, we'd probably hear the constant chatter of her mind, will and emotions, each rambling on about many different things. Her conscience may sound like . . .

"What *do* I want to eat this morning? Is that lady looking at me? I think CSI comes on tonight. You really ought to get the breakfast croissant . . . it's the best value. But what am I in the mood for . . . what am I really going to enjoy? That guy really needs a haircut. And where did he get those shorts? Stacey is going to kill me if I get to work late again. Why doesn't somebody else come to the counter to take my order? I'm really hungry!"

In this scenario, Mary is conscious of "self," which is her flesh. And . . . *those who are living the life of the flesh [catering to the appetites and impulses of their carnal nature] cannot please or satisfy God, or be acceptable to Him* (Romans 8:8 AMP). This kind of living is anything but peaceful.

Scenario 2: "Moral Restraint"
Let's say Mary has learned some principles of healthy living. She knows the consequences of making wrong choices and desperately wants to make right ones, but it is definitely a struggle. Her conscience acts as a voice of restraint, saying things like . . .

"Boy, that looks delicious, but I really shouldn't have it. Too many calories. Okay, I need something with whole grains, but I'm not eating oatmeal. Yuck! How can anybody eat that stuff? Look at her . . . she can eat anything she wants cause she's so thin. Why didn't God give me a metabolism like that? It's so unfair. Hey, I did take the stairs three days in a row last week, and I am drinking diet soda. Maybe I can splurge and get . . . What? It has how many calories? Great! It looks like I'm stuck with oatmeal!"

In this scenario, Mary is conscious of "the law." In other words, she knows a number of things that are good for her but has an even greater awareness of what is bad for her. Consequently, she is primarily drawn to the wrong foods. Interestingly, the Scripture says, *And all who depend on the Law [who are seeking to be justified by obedience to the Law of rituals] are under a curse and doomed to disappointment and destruction . . .* (Galatians 3:10 AMP). A life under "the law" is not a life of peace.

Scenario 3: "The Umpire of Peace"

Mary has matured in her commitment and now, along with her knowledge of what foods are good for her and the things she needs to avoid, she is also conscious of the calm and peace directing her from within her spirit. Listening to her conscience may sound like . . .

"I'm so grateful for the opportunity to eat and the wisdom to make good choices. I am committed to eating well, so I want to keep the calories under 250. Oh look, a new wrap, and it's only 225 calories. I've never tried anything like that before; it doesn't sound like anything I would like, but I really don't see anything else that will work. I'll try it. Wow! What a unique flavor. I never would have ordered this normally; I didn't even know I liked this kind of cheese. Thank You, Lord, for directing my choice and for a new-found delight."

In this last scenario, Mary is conscious of "the umpire of peace" living in her spirit. Colossians 3:15 gives us an excellent litmus test to help us make our decisions:

> *And let the **peace** (soul harmony which comes)*
> *from Christ rule (**act as umpire continually**)*
> *in your hearts [deciding and settling with*
> *finality all questions that arise in your minds,*

in that peaceful state] to which as [members of Christ's] one body you were also called [to live]. And be thankful (appreciative), [giving praise to God always].

—Colossians 3:15 AMP

What does it mean to let peace rule *as an umpire?* Well, think of the umpire's role in a baseball game. His eyes are glued to the action. He calls the plays and balls as he sees them, and his decision is *final.* In our lives, peace is the umpire, and its word is final. If we have peace about doing something, we can proceed—it's a "fair ball." If we don't have peace about something, we shouldn't do it—it's "out." Learning to follow after peace in all of our choices will enable us to experience a life of peace more and more.

> "The moment you wake up each morning, all your wishes and hopes for the day rush at you like wild animals. And the first job each morning consists in shoving it all back; in listening to that other voice, taking that other point of view, letting that other, larger, stronger, quieter life come flowing in."
> —C. S. Lewis[3]

LET HIM HAVE THE LAST WORD

Living a life of peace begins and continues through a life of surrender—turning yourself over to God and following His still, small voice moment by moment, day by day. Does this mean you should never listen to what your body is telling you or what your soul has to say about a situation? No. God has given you your mind, will, emotions and five senses for a reason, and there is a definite time and place for receiving their input. But He doesn't want you dominated by their voices or controlled by their cravings. Instead, He wants His Spirit, who lives in our spirit, to have the first and last word on the decisions we make. That's peace.

Keep in mind, a life of peace is not something you can achieve instantly; it is a *process learned through practice.* So continue to surrender yourself to God and receive His peaceful input in all your choices, including what you eat, how you play and the things you do day-by-day. Don't live in regret over the past or worry and fear over the future. *Give your entire attention to what God is doing right now, and don't get worked up about what may or may not happen tomorrow. God will help you deal with whatever hard things come up when the time comes* (Matthew 6:34 The Message).

HEART OF THE MATTER: *God granting our request* means experiencing **a life of peace**. This comes from learning to rest in Him, hearing and heeding the still, small voice of His Spirit living in our spirit over the constant chatter of our soul and body.

Recommended Resources: *Meditation for Christians: Experiencing the presence of God* by James Finley

(1) Definition of *Consciousness* (http://www.merriam-webster.com/dictionary/consciousness; retrieved 9-16-09). (2) Oswald Chambers, *My Utmost for His Highest* (Uhrichsville, OH: Barbour Publishing, Inc., MCMXCVII) p.232. (3) *Fast Break, Five-Minute Devotions to Start Your Day* (San Luis Obispo, CA: Parable, 2007) Day 33.

CONCLUSION

CONCLUSION

You Can Do It!

But thanks be to God,
Who gives us the victory [making us
conquerors] through our Lord Jesus Christ.

—1 Corinthians 15:57 AMP

God desires to prosper you on every level of your life, including
your health. He is all about you being healthy and whole—
spirit, soul *and* **body**. In Exodus 15:26, He is called Jehovah
Rapha, *the LORD who* **heals** *you* (NLT). Psalm 107:20 says,
He sends forth His word and **heals** *them and rescues them from*

the pit and destruction (AMP). And Psalm 103:3 declares He is a God *Who forgives [every one of] all your iniquities, Who* **heals** *[each one of] all your diseases . . .* (AMP).

Regardless of what other people say or how you feel or what you think, *you can do it!* You can lose weight in a healthy way and begin to see your entire life miraculously turned around by the mighty hand of God at work in you! Let's take a moment and recap what we've learned.

THE SEVEN POWERFUL PRINCIPLES OUTLINED IN THE PRAYER OF JABEZ

1   To find the answers you need to lose weight in a healthy way, *turn yourself over to God. Trust* in the wisdom of His 99%. Lean into life as a *"learner"* and expect amazing things to occur in your life.

2   As you begin to expand the way you look at your body, your life will be *blessed indeed!* In the process of living a new lifestyle, changes will appear in all areas, helping reinforce that you are staying out of TROUBLE. And the greatest blessing of all is the person you will become in the process!

3   The more blessed you become, the more God *enlarges your territory.* This means He "increases, expands and broadens" your opportunities on *every* level of life —physically, mentally, emotionally, spiritually, socially,

etc. Appreciate your success, your increased energy and the new way of doing things in your life.

4   As you apply the Seven Healers in your life you will begin to experience the *hand of God guiding you*. His hand is seen by your body's positive response to the things it needs most—*Air, Water, Sleep, Food, Play, Relationships* and *Purpose*. Look within and appreciate the "gospel of your body" by remaining sensitive to the wonderful changes you begin to experience.

5   *Keeping yourself from evil* means turning to God in prayer the moment you come to a crisis point. When the stress of any situation begins to overwhelm you, pray and ask God for wisdom to know how to honor your commitment and new way of living, as well as His grace not to give into old patterns of behavior.

6   Being overweight or obese *causes pain* to us and others, primarily because it keeps us from being able to participate in their lives in a meaningful way. In order to *not cause pain*, we must receive God's grace and the support of others to consistently *make right choices*.

7   *God granting our request* means we experience *a life of peace*. This comes from learning to rest in Him, hearing and heeding the still, small voice of His Spirit over the constant chatter of our soul and body.

Once you experience a certain level of success losing weight the Jabez way, you can begin to apply these same principles to many other areas of your life where stress exists, including your job, your finances, your marriage and your relationships with others.

For every child of God defeats this evil world,
and we achieve this victory through our faith.

—1 John 5:4 NLT

ONE MAN'S STORY OF VICTORY

To a great degree, *Weight Loss the Jabez Way* is about experiencing victory over aging and disease. These timeless principles were discovered and put into practice by a man I have personally known over forty years. Several years ago he found himself overweight and out of shape. After a routine trip to his doctor, he was told he needed to do something to lose some weight in order to regain the quality of life he had lost.

The first thing he began was walking with his wife. Sadly, this turned out to be a big disappointment and an even greater embarrassment because he couldn't keep up with her.

Ironically, not long after that, a close friend asked him to run a marathon. Knowing he couldn't keep up with his wife and his knee was giving him problems, he made a trip to his orthopedic doctor to get his opinion. An x-ray of his knee was taken, and it showed that it was in the same condition as an eighty-year-old man's due to a previous injury. With the glowing results hanging from the light box on the wall, the doctor said, "No, you can't run. You're just not going to make it with an eighty-year-old knee."

Deeply disappointed, the man responded, "So what will happen if I *try* to run?" The doctor replied, "You'll just end up getting the knee replaced earlier." Posing another question, the man asked, "So the worst thing that can happen is I will run the race, wear my knee out and have to have it replaced sooner, correct? I mean, I'm going to have to have it replaced anyway, right?" The doctor answered, "That's right." The man said, "Okay. Thanks, Doc," and off he went.

The next day the man went out and began running with two others, training for the marathon he had been invited to run. Now, it had been about 25 years since he had run, so he was grossly out of shape. He was totally unable to keep up with the others, and he became very discouraged. He cried to God in prayer saying, "Lord, I can't do this. There is no way I can run a mile, let alone this marathon. Who am I kidding? I can't even keep up with my wife when she walks. My knee is too old, I'm gasping for air and my body just can't take it. But I can't keep living my life this way. So I'm turning this whole situation over to you."

Right around this time, he had picked up a copy of the book *The Prayer of Jabez* and started reading it and praying the prayer while he was running. Every time doubts, fears and self-criticism came against him, he would pray the prayer, repeating it again and again and again. After turning to God and surrendering himself and the situation in prayer, he was able to break free from the limitations of the "1%" of what he knew and move into God's "99%" realm of the miraculous.

Little by little, his running time improved, he lost weight and he began to feel better than he had in years. The results were phenomenal! He not only ran one marathon, he ran *three*! And as of this writing, he is scheduled to run the New York Marathon in the fall. Without question, this man's life has been changed forever by the power of this prayer and the application of these principles. He and those close to him will never be the same. How am I so confident of this? Because *I am that man*!

> "Our greatest weakness lies in giving up.
> The most certain way to succeed is always
> to try just one more time."
>
> —Thomas Edison[1]

IT'S YOUR TURN!

Don't let the voice in your head or the discouragement of the devil drag you down. And don't listen to the negative naysayers who claim you'll never make it! With God, *all things* are possible, and you can do *all things* through Christ who strengthens you! (See Matthew 19:26; Philippians 4:13.)

Your answer to losing weight in a healthy way and keeping it off is not about buying another diet book or scouring the Internet for the latest and greatest methods of weight loss. It's really about coming to the end of yourself and the beginning of God. He is the Source of all wisdom and power. As you surrender to Him, apply these seven principles and stay in your commitment, *believe* you are changing, because you are! According to 2 Corinthians 3:18:

> *And all of us . . . are **constantly being**
> **transfigured into His very own image** in
> ever increasing splendor and from one degree
> of glory to another; [for this comes] from the
> Lord [Who is] the Spirit.* (AMP)

If God is living in you, *you are changing!* Little by little, from one degree to another He is doing a wonderful work in you. Cooperate with Him—passionately face and embrace the changes He is asking you to make. And by all means, smile, laugh and have fun with it! According to Proverbs 17:22, a light heart that is filled with laughter is mighty medicine. *And I am convinced and sure of this very thing, that He Who began a good work in you will continue until the day of Jesus Christ [right up to the time of His return], developing [that good work] and perfecting and bringing it to full completion in you!* (Philippians 1:6 AMP).

(1) Joyce Meyer, *Never Give Up!* (New York, NY: FaithWords, 2009) p. 109.